Marathon Method

I0161158

# Essential Guide to Training for Your First Half-Marathon

Selecting, training, and finishing
your first half-marathon the easy way

**JOE DONOVAN**

JULIANJOHN

Cover Design by Sean O'Connor
OhSeeDesign.com

**Special Note**: This edition of *"Marathon Method, Essential Guide to Training for Your First Half-Marathon"* is designed to provide information and motivation to our readers. It is sold with the understanding, that the publisher is not engaged to render any type of medical, psychological, legal, or any other kind of professional advice. No warranties or guarantees are expressed or implied by the publisher's choice to include any of the content in this volume. Neither the publisher nor the author shall be liable for any physical, psychological, emotional, financial, or commercial damages, including, but not limited to special, incidental, consequential or other damages. Before beginning any fitness or training program, consult with a medical professional.

Printed in the United States of America

# TABLE OF CONTENTS

Chapter                Page

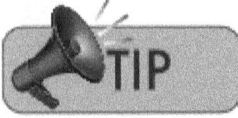

Throughout this book, you'll often see the TIP icon on the left. This book is filled with tips — the ones written next to this icon are those which I think are especially important. That said, I will now offer the best advice I can provide: Before you start any exercise program, including training for a half-marathon, it is critical that you get a check-up from your health care provider. I don't care if you are young or old, in shape or not, make an appointment with a qualified medical professional to ensure you are healthy enough to train and to be a long-distance runner.

This is important!

# PREFACE

As someone who has run multiple marathons, I know that few experiences match the feeling of crossing the finish line after months of preparation and training.

I stand firm that anyone can run a full marathon if they set their mind to it. However, it's a challenge that can understandably be quite daunting for those just starting out. Because you've picked up this particular book, I'll assume that you'd like to conquer the half-marathon before potentially moving on to run longer distances, A half-marathon is a lofty, yet attainable, goal that cuts back on a lot of the agony that comes with running a full marathon.

However, running a half-marathon is no easy feat, either, and those who finish one feel the same sense of accomplishment as their 26.2-mile counterparts. After all, the overarching goal is to become physically, mentally, emotionally, and spiritually healthier, and training for a half-marathon is a sure way to make great strides toward that achievement.

For many, the decision to participate in long-distance running comes after a major life-changing event, such as retirement, the birth of a child, or the death of a close friend or family member, or it's simply the result of a decision to approach life with a new and improved attitude. For others, it signifies the beginning of a new, healthier lifestyle, replacing former bad habits with more positive ones. But most importantly, long-distance running is about hope. In training for this challenge, there comes a certain hope that completing it will forever change your life for the better.

Of course, training for a half-marathon requires more than just hope. It requires preparation. This book will prepare you both mentally and physically for your first long-distance event. Think of it as a user's manual, complete with all of the tools, information, and motivation needed to accomplish your ultimate goal of crossing that finish line.

There are many books on the market that provide training methods for long-distance running, just as this one does. However, this book offers more, including how to begin your training, how to decide what gear to use, how to find the best half-marathon for you, important nutrition information, and numerous tips on how to prepare yourself for the challenge on all fronts.

While I strongly believe that anyone can master long-distance running, very few people actually make the commitment. Those who do consider the journey well worth their time and effort, often finding that they not only feel more energized and up-beat in their daily lives, but that they also have an improved sense of self, which benefits their lives, careers and relationships.

This book has one central theme: You <u>can</u> run a half-marathon. It may not seem like it right now, but you do have it in you.

I come to this assertion without ever meeting you or knowing anything about you. In fact, I have witnessed it countless times, having run with and coached thousands of people of all ages, shapes, sizes, and athletic abilities. Because of these experiences, I know that if you are healthy enough (make sure to check with your doctor) you can be a long-distance runner.

And so, if my encouragement has convinced you to run a half-marathon (and I sincerely hope that it has), I will promise you this – you'll get to that finish line.

Stick with me, and let's get started on your journey.

# 1: INTRODUCTION

> *"A lot of people run a race to see who's the fastest. I run to see who has the most guts."*
>
> - Steve Prefontaine

My personal desire to become a long-distance runner began when I was a kid, watching the New York City marathon on a Sunday morning sports TV show. From the view of a helicopter camera high above the Verranzano-Narrows Bridge, my brothers and I watched the runners make their way to the starting line, a scene which floored me beyond belief.

I couldn't believe that all of these people were going to try to run 26 miles—in a row!

I knew exactly how far 26 miles was, as the nearest McDonald's just happened to be about that far from our house. But I knew that if I tried to run there, they'd find me just down the block, collapsed on the side of the road. Running 26 miles was incomprehensible.

I wanted to watch every minute of the marathon, but my mother insisted that we eat breakfast and get ready for Sunday mass. When we returned from church, my brothers and I resumed our positions in front of the TV to watch the end of the race. We were glued to the screen as the winner made his final strides to the finish line, breaking the white tape with his arms raised in victory.

After that, a steady stream of runners followed suit, many of them celebrating their enormous accomplishment, even though they hadn't won the race. It was apparent that each of them had earned a personal victory.

As I watched the thousands of finishers, I said to my brother, "I could never run 26 miles." He paused for a moment before answering, not taking his eyes off the TV. We continued watching the runners on the screen—people of all shapes, sizes and ages—crossing the finish line. "You'd be surprised what you can do once you set your mind to it," he said.

I decided right then and there that I would someday run a marathon.

As it turned out, that "someday" was 19 years later, as I ran up the small Central Park hill that hid the finish line. Making my approach, the roar of the crowd grew louder and louder as the road narrowed between two sets of grandstands. I could hear an announcer's voice over a loudspeaker. As the crowd cheered and I spotted my friends and loved ones, I soaked in the magnitude of the moment.

I had finished a marathon. Not only that, but I had accomplished my goal of becoming a successful long-distance runner. For the first time in my life, I had set a long-term goal and really followed through with it.

With the finish line in sight, I was overwhelmed by a tremendous feeling of pride and accomplishment. I felt amazing. In fact, I felt like I could keep running forever. At that moment, anything seemed possible, as if everything that had ever gotten in the way of my dreams no longer mattered. As I would later find out, that feeling was there to stay.

I was nowhere near the front of the pack. In fact, by the time I finished, the winners had probably finished and enjoyed a solid meal. But I wasn't near the end, either. I finished right in the middle, and I couldn't have been happier with the result.

The day I finished my first marathon, along with my wedding and the births of my three children, was one of the best days of my life. Although I knew that being a long-distance runner would change my life, I had no idea that it would do so to such a great degree.

You see, once you complete a long-distance race, you start to feel like you have complete control over the other aspects of your life. And in many ways, you do. Many people satisfy their goals and desires by telling themselves that someday they will give it a shot, much like I used to. I used to let things happen to me, instead of making things happen. Running changed that.

Through your training for your half-marathon, you'll not only find that you will become healthier physically, but also mentally and emotionally. Things will start to become clearer, you'll be more active and aware, and you'll have much more energy and enthusiasm completing everyday tasks.

Personally, I learned that I am in charge of my own destiny and that life is too short to put off my goals. Since becoming a long-distance runner, I've received my Master's degree and have started my own business. I am now a husband and the father of three beautiful children. Since then, I have run in numerous marathons and long-distance events, including a triathlon and a long-distance mountain bike race. I have much more confidence than I've ever had, and I feel that I am in complete control of my life and what happens to me.

Above all else, I have learned one universal truth: With the proper health, time, and desire, *anyone* can be a successful long-distance runner.

My particular journey to the finish line was not especially unique or challenging. But to me, it was the one major event that I can look back on and honestly say that it truly changed my life. Starting out as a stressed-out and overweight office worker, I overcame barriers that sometimes seemed insurmountable. But I did it, and so can you.

Consider this book a user's manual to running your first half-marathon. For the most part, it is a how-to guide, complete with information on how to select and enter your first half-marathon, what gear and nutrition information you'll need, and how to take care of your body as it adjusts to changes and the demands of increased physical activity. I'll also give you some tips and effective "mind game" techniques which I have found helpful over the years. In this book, you'll also find a simple and effective training schedule, providing you with an easy-to-follow routine that will properly condition you for your half-marathon.

However, I hope you also benefit from more than just the logistics of the running program itself. If you're like me, your first half-marathon is more than just a race—it's a mission. I hope to inspire your mission by giving you a detailed account of the positive impact this challenge will have on your life.

I know you will accomplish your goal, and I want to help you every step of the way.

# 2: CONSIDERING THE HALF-MARATHON

> *"If you believe it's too difficult, it will be. If you believe it's possible, it will be. If you want it to be, you need to believe"*
>
> - Colin Mathieson

Half-marathons are gaining in popularity around the world. In fact, the number of runners participating in half-marathons has been increasing at a far greater rate than those running full marathons. And while many of us associate the word "marathon" with 26.2 miles, it's important to realize that the ability to run even 13.1 miles is something that only a small portion of us can do.

A half-marathon may be a better choice for you for a variety of reasons. First, and most obvious, it's less distance, which means less strain on the body and a less-intense training schedule. However, I must warn you that the conditioning will still likely be much more than you're used to, so be sure to get a check-up and take the necessary precautions before you begin.

Another reason for choosing a half-marathon may be that it will serve as an important benchmark on your way to eventually running a full marathon. After all, if you can finish a half-marathon, an impressive feat on its own, you'll know that you're capable of pushing yourself even further in the years to come.

Above all else, remember that a half-marathon is still a marathon in every sense of the word. Always keep in mind that what you're striving to achieve is extraordinary and the ultimate feeling you'll have when you have followed through with the goal that you have set for yourself is phenomenal.

Many, many people seriously consider long-distance running and think of completing a half-marathon as a secret goal. For some, the motivation is simply to become more fit, which is enough for them to strap on their running shoes and start training immediately. For others, as it was for me, a marathon is something to accomplish sometime down the road, when the time is right. At some point, though, we must make the commitment to dig in our heels and go for it.

In speaking with long-distance runners about how they got started, the issue of timing frequently comes up. For many new runners, a life-changing event is the final push they need to actually sign up and start training. I can't tell you how many people I've met who have beat cancer and decided to celebrate by running a marathon. Just think, at one point in their lives these people were next to death, only to bounce back and conquer one of the world's greatest physical challenges.

For a lot of people, like me, it's simply about making a lifestyle change to become healthier. Prior to my first marathon, I was an overweight and overworked aide in a U.S. Senator's office. I was getting married soon, and my fiancée and I wanted to start our family right away. With this major life change, I wanted to follow through on a promise I had made to myself years earlier. Whether the event in your life was positive (birth of a child, graduation of a child) or perhaps not-so-positive (divorce, death of a loved one), running a half-marathon can be an excellent way to use your energy to turn a new page in your life.

As it turned out, running a marathon made an unbelievably positive impact on my life—mentally, emotionally, and spiritually—with my only regret being that I had not done it earlier. From that, I offer this advice: If you want to become a long-distance runner and have the time, health, and the wherewithal to do it, start now. Don't wait until next month, next spring, or next year. Do it now.

## Committing to the Half-Marathon

There's no doubt about it, I believe that any healthy person can complete a half-marathon, as long as he or she has the time and the desire to do so. Think of it as a series of steps, whereas each individual step brings you that much closer to your goal. The program in this book outlines incremental steps over time that seem fairly easy, but you must be sure to not skip any of the steps. Doing so will only harm your conditioning progress and could set off a domino effect that could derail your training program.

You may find this hard to believe, but training for a half-marathon requires a lot of running. Week by week, the amount will vary, but you should expect to spend between a half hour and 45 minutes per weekday and several hours on the weekends preparing and training. Don't become overwhelmed by the amount of time you'll have to invest, because we'll start slow and work our way up. Just keep in mind that training does take time.

Long-distance running is also an added expense to your budget. As I will discuss in greater detail later, you don't need to spend a fortune on the best apparel and equipment, but there is a cost for extra shoes, clothing, entry fees, and travel expenses, especially if your half-marathon is in another state.

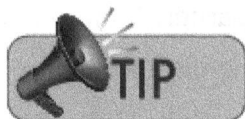

Here's a Tip! Training for distance running takes time, and there are expenses. If you don't have the time to progress through the entire program or the extra cash for the right equipment, wait till you do.

## Addressing the Skeptics

You may be surprised to find that loved ones will not always immediately understand your desire to run a half-marathon. Remember, it's not only you who is making the commitment, but also your partner or spouse, your children, and any other people who will be affected by the change in your schedule due to your training program. It is very important to discuss your plans with those close to you before you decide to complete your half-marathon. Be honest in explaining the time it will take to train and the added expense involved, but let them know that it is important to you.

You should also be honest in explaining the reason(s) you want to start long-distance running. If running a half-marathon is a lifelong dream or part of a commitment to get in shape and live a healthier lifestyle, tell them why it means so much to you. If they understand how important this is to you and why, they'll support you and celebrate with you.

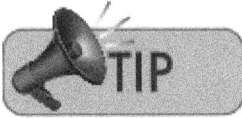

Here's a Tip! If you have kids, talk with them about the half-marathon. Use your experience as a way to teach your children the importance of setting and reaching goals. Sit down with your children and discuss what the half-marathon means to you and what kind of commitment it will take, on your part and theirs.

Once you've had a check-up, have discussed the commitment with your friends and family, and have considered the extra time and expense, you should be ready to take on the half-marathon challenge. Are you still with me? If so, let's get started.

# 3: THE FIRST STEPS

> *"The obsession with running is really an obsession with the potential for more and more life."*
>
> - George Sheehan

Now that you've decided to make the commitment to run a half-marathon, you're ready to take the first few steps toward your goal. Congratulations, you're on your way!

This chapter will provide you with information on how to take those next steps. Like most people, you're probably anxious to get started and feel like skipping this section of the book. Believe me, I know where you're coming from, but please hang in there. This section asks you to consider some important questions—thing that will help you later on.

Let's begin with determining the time frame for your half-marathon training.

## Marathon Time Frame

Completing a half-marathon takes a lot of planning and preparation, and it is very important that you give yourself enough time to fully prepare for it.

One of the most important aspects of training for long-distance running is establishing a solid running base. This may take awhile, and it's important to give yourself enough time in order to complete the 12-week running program in this book without a problem. For most people, eight months is enough time to complete the process.

Once they've conquered their first half-marathon, many runners decide to stay on a cycle of one event per year, or one every other year. This helps runners stay on track with their training and allows for them to continuously stay focused on a specific goal. My routine is to find an event far ahead of time and set up my complete training schedule before I begin on day one. I usually keep a calendar on my computer and diligently mark off the days until the race.

Keep in mind that this time frame is not written in stone. Like I said previously, most runners will be able to properly train in eight months time. However, for others, this will take a little longer. Be sure to talk with your health care provider and ask for his or her advice in regard to the conditioning time frame recommended for you. Above all, do not rush the process. Too many people fall short of running their half-marathon because they try to accomplish too much in too little time.

Remember, oftentimes the first steps involve smaller goals, such as losing weight, becoming more active and physically fit, or developing healthier eating habits. If you need to do this before embarking on your formal 12-week training program, that's not a problem. In fact, it will help you in the long run. Just give yourself plenty of time and stay on track. After all, you've given yourself eight months and you have plenty of time to get in shape, so don't feel like you're lagging behind just because you're not running multiple miles right off the bat.

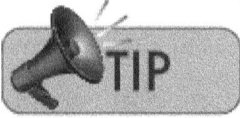

Here's a Tip! When you do decide what half-marathon to run, set an "official" start date for your training. Put it on your calendar and do something special to recognize the date. I like to have a special, "Start of Half-Marathon Training" run. When you set a start date, it's more difficult to postpone your training.

## Selecting Your Half-Marathon

As mentioned earlier, the number of people participating in half-marathons has steadily increased at a tremendous rate over the past several years. Likewise, the scope and prestige of various half-marathons across the United States (and the world, for that matter) has grown steadily. However, while the distance of 13.1 miles (about 21.1 kilometers) is always the same, the differences between races can be significant.

The sizes and difficulties of different half-marathons differ, depending on the location. The largest and perhaps the most famous half-marathon in the United States is the OneAmerica 500 Festival Mini-Marathon, run each year in Indianapolis, with a section of the course running right through the Indianapolis Motor Speedway, the site of the Indy 500. Recently, the number of runners has reached over 35,000, about the same amount that run the New York City Marathon each year.

Keep in mind that some of the larger half-marathons, like the OneAmerica 500, are so popular that not everyone is allowed to participate. This race is always sure to be a sellout, so you will need to register months in advance if you want to secure a spot at the starting line.

Another well-known race, the 3M Half Marathon, takes place in Austin, Texas in January and is mostly downhill. This event is often considered very friendly to first-time half-marathon runners.

Other notable half-marathons include the Colonial Half Marathon in Williamsburg, Virginia; the Chicago Half Marathon; the Walt Disney World Half Marathon in Orlando, Florida; and the Manhattan Half Marathon in New York City.

There are literally hundreds of half-marathon events scattered across the country, so if you're looking for one close to where you live, you'll likely find one sometime during the course of the year. Smaller events are nice because they give runners lots of individual attention and tend to be less formal. These half-marathons also often allow you to register right before the start. Choosing a smaller event because it's close by can be an advantage because it will allow you to train on the actual race course.

I have known many runners who prefer smaller events, for a variety of reasons. The most important thing is chose the half-marathon that's right for you and go with it.

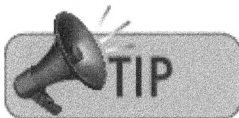

Here's a Tip! There are lots of things that must be considered when selecting a half-marathon, but here's a suggestion I'd like to share: Consider the possibility of traveling to a different city or part of the country to run your half marathon. For me, part of the adventure is being able to run in another city.

So, what marathon is best for you? While location is most likely one of the most important factors, there are also several other things to seriously consider.

As I noted, the Austin 3M Half Marathon is popular due to its downhill course. If the race you're considering is hilly, you may want to avoid it your first time out, unless you're used to training on hilly terrain. While many people do it, running a half-marathon on a hilly course adds an extra layer of complication to an already challenging run.

You should also think about when the event will be held. Long-distance events like these can take place during any season, and some areas with warm climates hold events in the middle of winter. While you should think about the conditions in which you'll run the actual half-marathon, you should also consider the type of weather in which you'll be doing a majority of your training. If you live in an area with cold winters, keep in mind that a spring half-marathon will require you to log a lot of long runs in cold weather. If you like the cold, then there's no problem. But if you're like me and hate running in cold weather, you might want to consider a fall event so you can train during the summer.

In addition, it's best to train in conditions similar to those in which you'll run your race. The summer months tend to provide weather similar to that in early fall, but the difference between winter and spring can be much more noticeable.

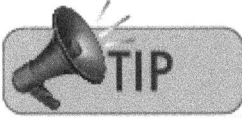

Here's a Tip! There are dozens of half-marathons around the country. For a comprehensive schedule of marathons worldwide, go to HalfMarathons.com.

## Registering for Your Half-Marathon

Regardless of which half-marathon you decide to run, make sure you review and become educated about the registration process and register as early as possible. Most events have a website where you can find out how to register, including deadlines, entry fees, race day procedures and other important information.

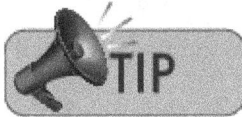

Here's another Tip! If you want to learn more about a particular half-marathon, you can always talk with someone who has already run it. Ask about the course, the crowd and whether there was enough water along the course and restrooms at the start and finish lines.

# 4: GETTING INTO GEAR

> *"No doubt a brain and some shoes are essential for marathon success, although if it comes down to a choice, pick the shoes. More people finish marathons with no brains than with no shoes.*
>
> - Don Kardong

One of the significant advantages of running long-distance events in this day and age is the dramatic improvements in shoes, running clothes, and nutritional supplements. As you start on your mission, make sure you have the right gear for the long road ahead. It's time to look at the most important pieces of equipment you'll need.

### Shoes

Not surprisingly, the most important single piece of gear is your shoes. Having good-fitting running shoes is critical, and trying to save a few bucks by scrimping on shoes is not a good idea.

That said, finding the right shoes for your feet is really difficult. There are so many different brands and models that it can be mindboggling and paralyzing. To get your head around finding the right shoes, it is important that you start with the right store.

Where do you go for help? Regardless of their size, most cities have a locally owned hole-in-the-wall running shoe store that is owned and employed by runners. This is where you want to buy your shoes. Not only will you get fitted properly in these stores, but you'll also be taken care of by fellow runners who have been on their own marathon mission.

For the last 15 years, I have driven more than an hour to a small shoe store where the people measure my feet and expertly fit me with the perfect shoes. Sure, a pair of shoes at this tiny store costs a little more than if I went to the mall or purchased them online, but the service I receive is well worth the extra cost.

These stores are often hard to find. The best way to find your area's local runner's store is to ask fellow runners.

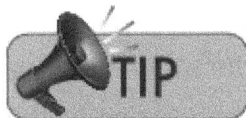

Here's a Tip! When you go to the store, you need to know that the right shoe for your foot might not be the best looking shoe in the store. In most cases, you can find a shoe that fits and meets modest demands for high fashion. But don't expect too much. Buy running shoes because they fit, not because they look good. Hey, we all want to look good. But do you want to know what is really ugly? Blisters. Enough said.

## Socks

The second most important piece of gear, in my opinion, is your socks. When I first started long-distance running, I wore basic white gym socks. What a mistake that was.

Regular old cotton gym socks are thicker than running socks and tend to hold onto moisture much more than a good pair of running socks. They are also much more likely to crease inside your shoe. Good running socks are lightweight, wick away moisture, and are much less likely to crease or have seams that cause blisters.

Blisters to long-distance runners are more than a pain — they can seriously wreck your training program. In most cases, blisters, especially serious blisters, can be avoided with good-fitting shoes and good socks.

I should point out that the high cost of a good pair of running socks may surprise you. All I can say is that it's worth it and they do tend to last a long time. You will thank me when you talk with a fellow runner who complains of blisters while you remain blister-free.

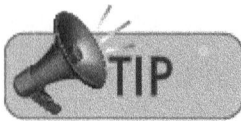

Here's a Tip! I like to wear the socks I'm going to wear in the race and in my training to the store when I buy my shoes. This ensures proper fit. I encourage you to do the same.

Two brands of socks that I highly recommend are WrightSock and SmartWool. The bad news is that good socks cost a lot of money. The good news is they last a long time.

### Shorts, Shirts, Tights

If at all possible, try to select the shorts and shirt you'll wear for your marathon early and wear them during your training. Sure, your neighbors might think you only own one set of running clothes, but what you give up in vanity, you'll make up for in knowing that you won't have a problem with your clothing when you're at the starting line.

I learned this the hard way. A few years ago, I needed a new running shirt. My old one, which had served me through hundreds of runs and two marathons, was looking pretty shoddy. I went to my local running store and, with great care, selected and purchased a new shirt.

It seemed exactly like my old one—same same manufacturer, same color, and same size—so I tried it out on my next long run. I found that I'd made a big mistake. While this shirt looked and felt exactly like my old one, the manufacturer had recently started treating their fabric with a new chemical that made the shirt reflective. It also made it very hot, especially during those last several miles. The lesson: Find clothes that work and stick with them.

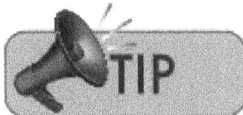

Here's a Tip! When you purchase shirts and shorts, take care to ensure the seams and tags are not going to cause problems. Getting back to the bounce factor, keep in mind that something as simple as a tag or a ill-positioned seam bouncing on wet skin for four hours will wreak havoc. I have seen men with bloody backs because of a tag and I've personally had broken skin due to a poorly fitting shirt.

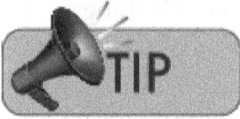

Here is another Tip! Keep in mind that the weather can change during your longer training runs and also during the marathon itself. Whenever possible, dress in layers that you can add to or shed as the temperature warms up and cools down.

## Support Items

It's hard to be subtle about this, so I'm just going to put it out there. Things bounce when you run — things that shouldn't bounce around, bounce around. Support is important.

As a former high school athlete, I recall a poster that was hung in the boys' locker room admonishing us to wear properly fitting athletic supporters. The poster said that failure to have the proper support would "result in irreversible damage." Now, I'm no health professional, but I do know that support is important.

So, when you're at the store, ask the salesperson to show you different types and brands of support gear. If you are a woman and your salesperson is a man, don't be afraid to ask if there is a female salesperson who can show you a bra. They won't be offended, and you shouldn't be ashamed. The same thing goes for a guy. Talk with someone who uses the same stuff you'll wear.

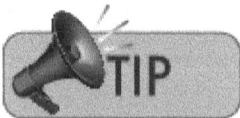

Here's a Tip! If it's uncomfortable in the store, it won't be comfortable when you run. Also, keep in mind you have to pay for comfort. Good-fitting support items are expensive.

## Hats, Watches, Sunglasses

I tend to do a lot of my longer runs along a paved trail that has become a favorite training place for other marathon runners. As a result, I tend to run with lots of other people who are training for various events. One of the mind games (I'll explain mind games in greater detail later) I use is to count the number of runners who are wearing hats. During my last ten years of running, I've noticed more and more people, especially women, wearing visors and hats.

I'm not a hat guy myself, but many people swear by them to keep themselves cool and to keep the sun off their faces. I also see a lot of people wearing sunglasses and watches. Here again, I don't run with either, but a lot of people do.

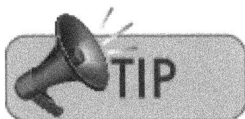 Here is a Tip! If you do wear a hat, sunglasses, a watch, a cape—whatever you wear—don't wait until you begin longer runs to start wearing it. Also, and I'll repeat this again later, if you wear a hat to train, wear it during the race. Find what works and stick with it.

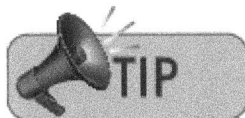 Here is another Tip! As I mentioned, I tend to do a lot of my running in the early morning and at night. Because my runs require that I cross a lot of city streets, I am always concerned that people driving cars can see me. Reflective gear helps, but I've found a better way to be seen. When I run, I carry in my hand a little LED light. It's made for putting on a bike, but because it is very small, it's easy to carry. It

is also extremely bright and can be set so it blinks. As I run, I carry it in my hand so it is facing traffic to make sure drivers see me. This is especially helpful when crossing dark intersections.

## To Jam or Not to Jam

If you run a course where there are a lot of other runners, you'll see that many of them listen to music, using an mp3 player and headphones. The decision to listen to music is an individual one and is totally up to you.

Personally, I'm not a big fan of listening to music when I run, but I know many runners who say that music keeps them pumped up during their runs. If you do decide to listen to music, make sure that both the audio player and the music itself is not a distraction. I recommend purchasing an armband to hold your mp3 player and creating a playlist that will last your entire run, so that you don't have to worry about manually changing songs.

# 5: MIND OVER MATTER

> *"Some of the world's greatest feats were accomplished by people not smart enough to know they were impossible."*
>
> - Doug Larson

By now, you've chosen your half-marathon, registered and have been accepted in it, and have started your training. The next step is a big one—getting your mind wrapped around the idea that you're going to complete a half-marathon and what it will take to get there. Make no mistake about it, this will be a big challenge, but it will be one that will take you from who you are today into a successful long-distance runner. If this is the first time in your life that you're getting into shape, this can be a hard concept to believe. But you'll get there, and this section of the book will discuss a crucial part of your preparation—training your mind.

## Pumping Yourself Up

There are many, many books available that outline the importance of self-talk and keeping a positive attitude. I encourage you to find as much information as you can to help you along your journey, but I'd also like to add three pieces of advice that have been critical to my success as a runner:

## (1) Don't let negative thoughts enter your mind.

This advice was given to me by a college professor, and it has stuck with me ever since. You've likely heard something like this before, but like me, haven't thought much about it. However, when pushing yourself to your personal limits, it's important to stay positive; focus only on positive things and never dwell on the negative. Let's face it, bad things happen to all of us every day, and you may feel a sense of negativity, especially as you grow tired toward the end of your runs. It's the ability to leave those negative thoughts behind you as you run that results in true success.

Let me be a little more specific and blunt. When I first started long-distance running, I was overweight. I hadn't done much running, I didn't have a great diet, and I wasn't exactly the picture of fitness. To me, the distance sometimes seemed insurmountable, and I didn't feel like I really knew what I was doing. If I would have focused on all of those obstacles, I never would have completed my goal.

However, staying positive can be easier said than done. Setting out to run a half-marathon is a calculated leap of faith, in that you're counting on your body, with the right preparation and training, to last 13 miles. It's natural to have doubts, which brings me to my next tip:

## (2) Don't be logical.

This is especially true if you're the type of person who must logically dissect everything in an attempt to make a clear decision in every situation. Generally, being logical and using common sense is (of course) a good thing, but with long-distance running, it can sometimes hinder your self-confidence. You have to be disciplined, not allowing yourself to think about why you can't do it, and only focusing your thoughts on why and how you will do it. Push out those negative thoughts and don't be logical.

**(3) View yourself as a marathoner.**

When you look back on it, you'll realize that the day you became a marathoner was not the day you crossed the finish line, but when you first *believed* that you could complete a half-marathon. When you're out on your conditioning runs, remind yourself that what you're doing is extraordinary and that you are on an important, life-changing mission. You are a long-distance runner and an <u>athlete</u>. Most people don't consider themselves to be athletic, but it's hard to argue that a person who can run 13.1 miles is not an athlete. You're an athlete. Doesn't that feel great?

## Sharing Your Goal

Now that you've started on the right path to keeping yourself upbeat about your half-marathon goal, it's time to tell as many people as you can about your mission (without being obnoxious). This is very important, because not only will it force you to discuss your training in a public setting, but it will hold you to it by making it more difficult to back out of it. Think of it as an extra layer of motivation. If people express disbelief in your goal or that you can complete it, use it as motivation to keep yourself on the right track.

When I started my training, I didn't look like a long-distance runner. I needed to shed a few pounds, and most people knew me as a nine-to-five office worker who was no stranger to junk food. One of the common perceptions out there is that runners have to be stick-thin running machines. However, I know I didn't look the part—and I still don't—at least not in the eyes of the people around me.

So, naturally, when I started telling people that I was going to start running and for long distances, I got a lot of odd looks. In some cases, I received an unenthusiastic "that's nice," with an obvious undertone of disbelief. Other times, when speaking with friends or co-workers, they'd take a step back, look me up and down and say, "You? *You* are going to run a marathon?"

Don't look at it as a setback if you get a similar response. Instead, use it as even more motivation to accomplish your goal. However, always remember that this journey is for you, and you have nothing to prove to the people around you.

In the end, you may find that the people who acted surprised when you first shared your half-marathon goal with them will turn out to be your most enthusiastic supporters. That's certainly what happened with me. It wasn't that they didn't believe in me, they were just surprised that I, someone who they'd least expect, was going to be a long-distance runner.

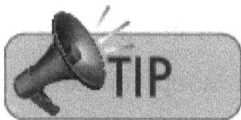 Here's a Tip! While you can run a half-marathon and not tell anyone about it, I think half the fun, especially for your first event, is in sharing your goal with other people. Be an inspiration to others.

Try to make your half-marathon a conversation piece. Don't overdo it, but let those around you know what you're up to and how important it is to you. They'll likely ask about your progress from time to time; don't be afraid to share your accomplishments and the challenges you encounter along the way. As people watch you make progress in your training, their interest will grow, and so will their support. They'll also notice your change in attitude, as your new and heightened confidence will inevitably have a positive effect on your everyday demeanor. Enjoy this feeling – it's why you've made the half-marathon your mission in the first place!

The bottom line is to do yourself a favor and tell people about your goals, but don't get too disappointed if their reactions are different than what you expected.

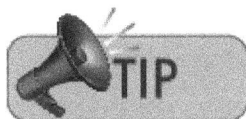 Here's a Tip! You will receive lots of positive comments from friends about your half-marathon plans. Take mental stock of these comments. I encourage you to keep a running list of people who share your excitement about the race; these are people you can call for encouragement and to share the good news with when you finish.

## You are a Machine

One of the great things about long-distance running is that you will start to truly understand how your body works. You'll find out its limits, which foods make it work best, and the best way to recuperate from small aches and pains. Basically, you'll realize that your body is a machine.

During your training, you will be asking your body to do things it has never done before. It may sound cliché, but your body is going to need a healthy diet and plenty of rest to adapt to your increased physical activity.

Training for a half-marathon will make you aware of the downside of eating the wrong foods and failing to get enough sleep. A long night of beer and onion rings before a long run simply won't work. Relying on your body to get you through those long runs will force you to make sure you put the right fuel in your tank and that you are getting enough sleep. That was a true wake-up call for me, and a lesson that has served me well since.

This step is one of the most positive ones you'll make in your marathon journey. I have seen lives change, almost overnight, as a result of people's changes in perceptions about their bodies. I have seen people, who were significantly overweight and hooked on fast food, start packing a healthy lunch, losing weight and keeping off those extra pounds. I have also seen people who have smoked most of their lives kick the habit for good.

These people knew that smoking and poor eating habits weren't good for them, but it was running that forced them to make a change. Neither fast food nor cigarettes go well with running, and success depends on dropping those bad habits.

Do you have any bad habits? If so, it's likely they won't mix well with your new training routine.

If you've made it this far in the book, you should already be proud of yourself. You're taking direct action to better your life, and that's something to be admired. Before moving on, take a moment to let this feeling sink in.

Now, let's start running.

# 6: RUNNING TO A SOLID FOUNDATION

> *"Running is a big question mark that's there each and every day. It asks: 'Are you going to be a wimp or are you going to be strong today?"*
>
> - Peter Maher

In my first *Marathon Method* book, which focused on the training program for running a full marathon, I laid out a multi-week "pre-program," or base-building section, the purpose of which was to get the body in better shape and ready for the actual training program. For a half-marathon, this is no different. Your 12-week program, which will be laid out in upcoming chapters, will be rigorous at times, so it's important to build a base you can use to prepare for some serious running.

If you ask anyone what the most difficult part of running a marathon is – full or half – and they'll tell you it's the first mile, not the last. As is the case with any long-term goal, the biggest challenge is getting started. In this section, we'll start off slow and get you pointed in the right direction.

When most people decide to start running, they are excited about their first run. They throw on their new gear, lace up their shoes, take their time stretching and warming up and energetically head out the door for the first time. In their minds, they envision a nice, easy jog—likely without the need to even stop for a breather. They embark down their chosen course with brisk, even strides.

Several minutes later, you'll often find them grabbing their sides, their hearts pumping out of their chests. That first run isn't going to go very well—in fact, it's not going to be much fun at all. Two blocks down the road, you are already going to feel winded, your legs will feel like boat anchors, and you'll have some serious doubts about ever running 13.1 miles.

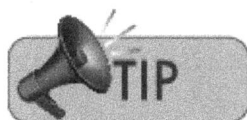

**Here's a Tip!** Remember what I said about negative self-talk? Don't do it. You should know that your first run is going to be very bad. Don't worry. I don't care if you only go 100 feet. You will run a half-marathon. Don't defeat yourself.

## Building Your Base

Most of the time, when referring to the training program for a half-marathon, we're referring to the 12-week rigidly specific schedule in the months leading up to your race. I've included that program later in this book, but before you start it, you need to get yourself into adequate shape to begin. The time frame for this pre-training is different for everyone, and only you will know when you're ready to move on. Few things can be more frustrating, and can derail your training more quickly, than not being fit enough when you begin the process.

So, how can you tell when you're ready? If you've been running three to five days per week (eight to 12 miles a week), and can comfortably run three miles and have been doing this for six weeks, you are ready to begin your training program. If not, just give it time and adapt the pre-training program to fit your needs.

Because I don't know your current level of fitness, and this is generally a book for beginner-level runners, I'm going to assume that your fitness level is fairly low. That is, you're healthy enough for training (you did get that check-up, right?) but either you aren't running or haven't built up a solid base yet.

First things first, we're going to get you running. Then, once you've started to get comfortable with it, we're going to establish a good fitness base before we start the actual program. Creating this base is extremely important, as it will serve as the foundation for your training. If your foundation is strong, you'll find that it'll be much easier to build upon your base more quickly and easily.

Remember, the length of this pre-program will vary depending on the person. Don't get discouraged. Keep working until you achieve your base, and I promise you'll be ready.

## Getting Started

For the first couple of weeks, or whenever you are comfortable enough to move on, I want you to do something I call the run-walk. The key is to run for a few minutes and to walk for a few minutes. I think it works best when you run slowly and walk briskly. Keep in mind that you will be pushing yourself and may get winded, but you should not feel any pain. If you do, talk with your health care professional.

Also, I want you to know that while our 12-week training program will be very prescriptive, this part of the program isn't. Do what works for you with the goal of getting to a point when you can run for 30 minutes straight.

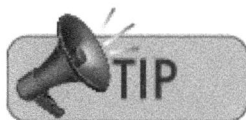

Here's a Tip! Stretch well. I find that most people have some knowledge of stretching and know that stretching is important. The problem is that most people simply don't do it. They should. Get in the habit of stretching each muscle group from your toes to your neck. In addition, stretching isn't something you should only do just before your run; it is also something you should do after your runs as part of your cool-down routine. As you will see, training for long-distance running is largely a set of routines. Do yourself a favor and make gentle and slow stretching a part of your routine. See the chapter on stretching for more information.

# Let's Get Started!

## Week One

Like I said, this week might be tough, but it'll get easier as you progress. For this week, simply try to run for one minute, then walk for five minutes and repeat the cycle three times. Do this three or four times the first week. Take it easy, run slowly, and don't push yourself too hard. Remember, you're just getting started and your body will need time to get used to the increased activity.

If this routine is too easy, try running for two minutes straight and walk for five. No matter what, keep your walking time at five minutes between mini-runs. This will give you more time to recuperate after each burst, and by walking, you're still getting exercise. Enjoy!

## Week Two

Once your one-minute runs become easy (hopefully in a week or so), bump it up to two minutes of running, then walk for five minutes, and repeat three times. Again, try to do this three or four times in a week.

How are you feeling? Make sure you are stretching properly and warming up before you go out, even though you're not going for full runs.

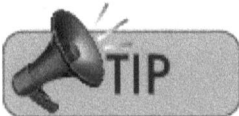 Here's a Tip! Use your breathing as your guide when running. You should be able to carry on a conversation while running, and your breathing shouldn't be heavy.

## Week Three

All right, we are on a roll. When you are ready (again, hopefully within a week), let's bump it up to running for four minutes and walking for three, repeating three times. Keep that up for four run-walks per week.

By this time, you might already feel better about yourself overall. Do you feel like you're in better shape than you were three weeks ago? Enjoy that feeling!

## Week Four

If you're following along and keeping up, you're doing well and are well on your way. This week, you are going to run for six minutes, keeping your walking time at three minutes and repeating twice. If you are feeling strong, repeat for a third time for a total of 24 minutes of solid running.

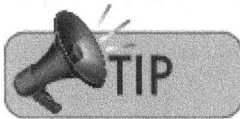

Here's a Tip! Drink water at the end of your workouts to rehydrate. If it's hot and humid, you should also drink some water (about 4 to 6 ounces) halfway through your workout.

## Week Five

Keep it up, you're doing great. This week, you will walk for two minutes and run for eight minutes. You will repeat this cycle three times, and do four sessions a week.

Are you hanging in there? Feeling good? Remember, run slowly and stretch well before and after your runs.

## Week Six

Let's turn it up a notch. This time after you stretch, you will walk for two minutes before running for nine minutes. Repeat this three times. Get four good sessions in this week. I encourage you to take a nice, long walk over the weekend. Wear the clothes you wear when you run, including your shoes, and try to walk for at least 45 minutes.

Aim to run for 30 minutes four times per week, and you'll notice your stamina and fitness will continue to improve.

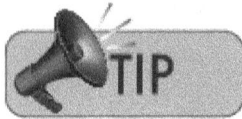

Here's a Tip! Now is a good time to join a local running club. Most large cities have a club that has training programs and classes for new runners. Not only are these clubs a great way to get started in running, but they are a great way to meet people.

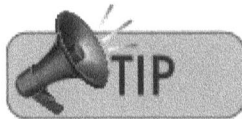

Here's another Tip! Take care in selecting who you run with. I'm not only talking about running with someone who runs the same distance and pace as you do, but also someone you are very comfortable with. There are some rather unglamorous facets of long-distance running. Burping and passing gas is sometimes inevitable, so make sure you are comfortable being seen at your worst in front of this person.

**TIP**

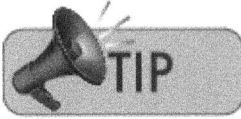

Here's another Tip! Prior to running a half-marathon, I think it is a good idea to run some local road races. In most parts of the country, these races or "fun runs" are plentiful. Not only is this a great way for you to experience a marathon on a much smaller level, but you get used to the lineup, running in crowds, and taking water while you are running.

# 7: FEED THE MACHINE. AVOID THE WALL.

> *"Too eat is a necessity, but to eat intelligently is an art."*
>
> - La Rochefoucauld

## The Wall

If you speak with enough long-distance runners, you may have heard them talk about hitting "the wall." While this term is most often used in the context of people who run or are training to run full marathons, it is certainly possible to hit the wall if you're running lesser distances. In order to avoid hitting the wall, you need to make sure you are giving your body the energy it needs through proper nutrition and diet, which I will help you with in this chapter.

"Hitting the wall" is the term runners associate with the experience of having severe muscle fatigue, which makes it difficult to run. In some cases, it can be simply that your muscles don't feel like they're working anymore. In others, it can include extreme dizziness, nausea, and confusion, among other more serious side effects.

Most runners I know have experienced the wall in some form or another, but their descriptions of the feeling vary. Personally, I've hit the wall a number of times and have felt more or less like I was dragging an extremely heavy object behind me as I ran. In most cases, I've run into the wall after failing to give my body enough fuel for a long run. Chances are you'll likely experience something similar to hitting the wall during your training, so it may take that experience for you to truly understand what I'm talking about.

Basically, the wall is the point where you've run out of energy. Scientifically speaking, it's a little more complicated, but I will do my best to explain it.

As you may be aware, our body's top energy source is carbohydrates, although we also burn fats. When you first start out running, your body gets about three-quarters of its energy from carbohydrates and the rest from fatty acids. However, as we progress in our long runs, we use up our carbohydrates and our bodies begin to burn more fatty acids.

This is why it's so important to get enough carbohydrates before you start out on your runs. If you get a sufficient amount in your system, you should have plenty to get you through even your long race-day run (a full 13 miles) without using up all of your stored carbohydrates.

Let's say you don't get enough carbohydrates before one of your long runs. After all of your calories in the form of carbohydrates are burned, you hit the wall and your body starts burning fat. Great, right? Well, not really. It doesn't work that way.

You see, your body doesn't have a lot of oxygen to help metabolize the fat, and so the burning of fat is much less efficient than the burning of carbohydrates. A by-product of this inefficient burning is lactic acid, and as a result, your legs essentially feel like they've turned to Jell-O.

So, how do you avoid the wall? The best advice I can give you is not to hit it in the first place by preparing yourself nutritionally. Also, make sure you are listening to your body and making sure you're giving it enough energy for your longer runs.

## Nutrition and Running

Nutrition is one of the most important topics to consider in your half-marathon preparation. The best training schedule in the world is worthless if the fuel you expect your body to run on is junk. However, I know that the topic of nutrition can be confusing and overwhelming. Let's go over the basics and hopefully you can take it from there based on the in-depth knowledge you have of your own body.

The simple basics of nutrition for the long-distance runner are that in order to be successful in your race, you must ensure that you remain well-hydrated and maintain an adequate supply of glucose. These two tips are very important for people engaging in any intense athletic activity, just as you are.

There are, of course, other nutritional items you should consider. Your body is a machine that requires fuel, and without this fuel, it won't run. With this in mind, it is important you pay careful attention to the foods you put into your body. You probably won't be surprised when I urge you to make sure you have adequate servings of fruits and vegetables. Also, make sure that you have plenty of protein in your diet. Personally, I'm not a big meat-eater, so I rely on eggs, beans, seafood, and (if I'm really hungry) soy. Of course, make sure you have plenty of carbohydrates in your diet. Fruits and vegetables are a good source of carbs, as are whole grains.

I tend to stay away from processed carbohydrates, like white bread. Instead, I try to eat things like wheat bread, sweet potatoes, and long grain rice. A good tip for bread is to look for products that do not contain enriched flour, which can be just as bad for you as sugar.

Over the years, there has been a lot of debate about how many of your calories should come from carbohydrates. Based on many conversations and my own experience, my rule of thumb is that 65% of your calories should come from carbs. Finally, try to stay away from high-fat foods, food with a lot of empty calories (like soda and candy) and any fried foods.

## Loading Up on Carbs

One of the more common questions I get from first-time runners is if they should "carbo-load" before a race, that is, if they should eat extra portions of carbohydrates in the days leading up to a long run or race.

The answer is yes. I advise new runners to begin carbo-loading two days before their long run or race to make sure their muscles store as much glycogen as possible. In practice, this means adding an extra portion of carbohydrates to every meal in your otherwise balanced diet. In addition, take in an extra glass of water because as the body increases its glycogen stores, it also increases the amount of stored water.

Immediately prior to a long training run or the event itself, I make sure I am well-hydrated. I also eat a light, but high-carbohydrate, meal no later than two hours before the race or run. And, by all means, take advantage of the water, sports drinks, and other glucose-containing foods that are often available at the aid stations.

You should also prepare for your long training runs the same way you prepare for the race for which you're training. Try to eat the same way you will eat the day of the marathon and also try to replicate when and what you will drink. Then, when it comes to the day of the half-marathon, you'll know what works and your body will expect what you're providing it.

In the week before your long runs and during the race itself, make sure you are well-hydrated. You are also carbo-loading at this time, so drinking water is best. Research has shown that carbohydrates convert to glycogen more effectively when accompanied with water. Also, choose foods for lunch and dinner that are high in carbohydrates (e.g., pasta, potatoes, rice, etc.). Don't neglect fruits, vegetables, ensure you consume some source of protein, and try to significantly scale back on fats during this time.

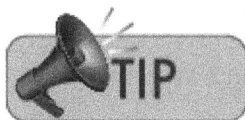

Here's a Tip! If you are traveling by plane to your marathon destination, carry bottled water with you. Flying at high altitudes causes dehydration.

## Give it Gel

One of the techniques that people use to ensure they keep enough fuel in the tank as they run is to consume sports gels. The most popular gel, and the one I am familiar with, is Power Gel made by Power Bar. Another popular brand is Gu.

The gels are available in many different flavors, the most popular being chocolate. Imagine really, really sweet cake frosting, and you have a sense of the taste and consistency of the gels.

The gels are packaged in small 40-gram foil containers that fit in the palm of your hand. Each gel foil packs a walloping punch of carbohydrate calories that are quickly absorbed by your system. There are many differences of opinion about using gels. It is important that you take the gels with water. If you don't have water, your body can't easily absorb the gel and you're likely to get sick. If you decide to use gels for your half-marathon, I would advise using one and taking it somewhere between mile eight and ten to give you that extra burst for the final few miles.

In following up with some people to whom I've recommended gels, I've learned some runners can benefit from them, while others find them unnecessary or problematic in that the sweet mixture sours their stomach. Give them a try during your training runs to see if they work for you.

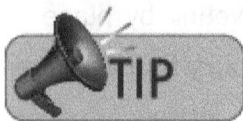

Here's a Tip! Once again, you should replicate what you've done in training when you are running your marathon. If you use gels while training, you should plan to use gels during your event.

## Water or Sports Drinks

Another question I've received from many people over the years is: Should I drink water or sports drinks? Here is a simple rule of thumb: In most cases, water should be your drink of choice. You should drink lots of water during the day for your general health, and you should drink water for all runs which last under 90 minutes.

Sports drinks, such as Gatorade, should be consumed for runs lasting over 90 minutes. I find my stomach has a hard time late in the race drinking straight Gatorade, so I tend to mix water and the sports drink. During my training runs, I dilute Gatorade with water and put it in a water bottle.

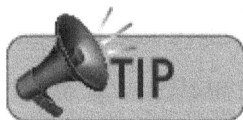

Here's a Tip! It is very important that you develop a good routine of drinking fluids while you run. Don't rely on your thirst mechanism to indicate signs of dehydration because it is very difficult to "catch up" on your fluid requirements if you are already dehydrated. You have to keep your fluids up by taking in fluids on a regular basis while you run.

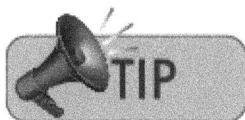

**TIP** Here's another Tip! When it comes to sports drinks, find out which brand and flavor will be distributed along the race course and use the exact kind and exact flavor when you train.

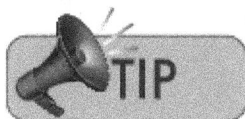

**TIP** Here's another Tip! You may have heard news stories about people who drink too much water while they run and have other problems. Yes, you can drink too much while you run. Don't go overboard by drinking excessive amounts of water or sports drink while you run; just drink enough to maintain good fluid levels.

During a race, I drink two sips of water every mile and add two sips of sports drink every other mile. If it's hotter, I drink more.

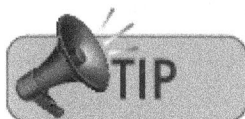

**TIP** Here's another Tip! Pay attention to the color of your urine. Generally, your urine should be clear with only a slightly yellow tint. Urine that is darker suggests you are dehydrated and need to drink more water.

# 8: MIND GAMES

> *"Mental attitude is 75 percent of winning."*
>
> - Vince Lombardi

The tired, old cliché that often comes with most athletic activity, regardless of what kind, is that the mental state of mind is always more important than physical ability. Growing up in Wisconsin, in the land of the Green Bay Packers where Vince Lombardi is legend, I often heard one of his famous quotes: "Mental attitude is 75 percent of winning."

Of course, variations of this quote, in both wording and percentage, are widespread in our culture. And like many famous quotes, this one is quite true. Only when it comes to long-distance running, I'll bump that percentage up to 90 percent. That is, 90 percent of preparing, training, and running a half-marathon rests in how you deal with the challenge in your head.

If you think about it, the physical aspect of running a half-marathon is quite easy. All you have to do is get up and run, and run often, and eventually you'll get there. It's the mental side of it that creates such a seemingly-enormous barrier for so many runners.

This chapter is all about what's going on in your head. I'll lay out some great tips I've learned over the years to train your mind as you train your body.

## Avoiding Monotony

As your body adjusts to your longer runs, you'll find that there will be a lot less of a physical toll on your body each time. Your body will recuperate faster and you won't feel completely winded after multiple miles, which will be a wonderful feeling. However, you may find another unexpected enemy—boredom.

When I first started running long distance, a more experienced runner told me that his mind tended to wear out before his body. I had no idea what he was talking about at the time, but as I became more physically fit, I started to understand. As my mileage increased, I found that my body was doing great, but I was having trouble dealing with the monotony of my long runs, not to mention the loneliness. While it was sometimes nice to get away from the pressures of my everyday life, I found that I was bored much of the time. I started to dread my longer runs for that reason alone.

However, over the years, I have found a great method to prepare for long runs that takes away a lot of the boredom I used to experience. In fact, now I almost always look forward to days when I embark on 10-plus milers.

The key to overcoming boredom is to concentrate on something. Before I start my long runs, I make a list of all of the things in my life that I need to sort out by the end of the week.

Then, when I'm on my run I can give each decision serious thought and come to a definite conclusion, not feeling like I rushed things. Whether it's a small decision (like where to take the family out to dinner next weekend) or a big one (like whether to make a risky investment), a long run can be a great time to really become deep in thought.

Because of this, your running time can be used as time in which you're also the most productive. In life, we're often forced to make difficult decisions without thinking them through, which can sometimes lead to negative consequences. One of the great by-products of training for long-distance running is that I often make good choices after completely considering all of the options.

You should also try to use your running time to relax. During the week, I make a deal with myself, promising not worry about certain things. Then, while I'm running, I use that time to worry about whatever happens to be bothering me. Beyond prompting action, worrying for the sake of worrying is not productive or beneficial, so I deal with my worries when I run. For a mile or two, I allow myself to think about what's been bothering me, but then I leave it behind as I run, both literally and figuratively. Try it. It works!

Above all else, I am sometimes surprised to find myself praying during my longer runs. It's surprising because I'm not usually the most spiritual person in the world, but there's something about the calming nature of running and the rhythmic sound of steps that allows me to think deeply about things that normally I don't or can't think much about.

By giving you this information, I hope you can avoid what I went through at first – a hatred of long runs. If you do some mental preparation, long runs can be a great time for personal and spiritual growth.

## Check Yourself

Although the tips above can be helpful, especially on longer runs, you should also make sure not to get too deep in thought, to the point where you're not paying attention to your surroundings or your body's needs.

To ensure that you don't become a running zombie, force yourself to do a quick "systems check" at every mile. Ask yourself if you feel any unusual pain, if you need food or water or need to take a bathroom break. On long runs, it can be easy to lose track of time and forget about what your body needs, especially if you're busy thinking about other things.

## Dealing with Pain

I owe it to you to be completely honest about this aspect of long-distance running: sometimes, it will hurt. There's not much you can do about it, as it is simply part of the process. If the pain becomes unbearable, check in with your healthcare provider, especially if you're experiencing an intense or sharp pain or if something just doesn't feel right.

One a day-to-day basis, there will be some aches and pains that you'll have to deal with. You'll find that at a certain point in your run, your legs will start to hurt, which will likely be more annoying than anything. What's important is that you don't let these pains sidetrack you. It's all part of being a long-distance runner, and eventually you'll get used to it. Your body is tough and will be able to work through the pain, as long as you keep your mind off the discomfort.

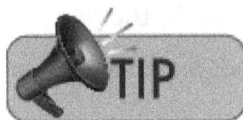

Here's a Tip! The way I deal with inevitable aches and pain while I am running is to welcome it. That's right. I force myself to think of the upcoming pain, like I am meeting up with an old friend who will run with me for a while. When I feel the aches beginning, I say to myself, "There you are old friend; how are you?" Then, I literally imagine myself running next to an old friend.

I know it seems strange. I felt that way when I heard this advice. But it works.

### Avoid the "Fog"

If you've spent time reading about running or talking with runners, you might have come across the concept of a "runner's high," or a feeling of euphoria after completing a long run or other strenuous activity. While I'm not sure that I've experienced the feeling as I've had it described to me, I do have a friend who swears that he can take on the world after he finishes a long run. All I know is that running makes me feel better mentally and physically, which is why I run in the first place.

One thing I have experienced many times is what I call the "runner's fog." A lot like daydreaming, the runner's fog is drifting into a state of mind where you stop thinking about running, although you continue to run. In other words, you get so deep in thought that you literally forget that you're running.

For me, I tend to be most apt to drifting into a fog when I run the same course again and again. There's something about the familiarity that makes me daydream.

Many runners I've talked to over the years love the feeling of the fog. They say it makes them feel more relaxed and allows them to get a long run in without experiencing some of the negative aspects of running. However, slipping into this state of mind can be a little dangerous.

As I mentioned, it's important to perform quick system checks to keep yourself alert. When you daydream while running, it's easy to forget your body's basic needs, like food and water. I've also found that in the fog, I make some poor decisions, like crossing streets without looking or tripping over cracks in the sidewalk.

The lesson is to find a healthy balance between using your running time to think about things and making sure that you're staying sharp during your run. Relax, but keep your mind active.

# 9: AVOIDING INJURY / STRETCHING

> *"I never struggled with injury because of my preparation - in particular my stretching."*
>
> - Edwin Moses, Olympic gold medalist

In many ways, this chapter is about prevention. For the next several pages, we will go over some techniques that will help you to prevent injury from derailing your half marathon mission. It would be unfortunate, not to mention frustrating, to have to delay your plans due to a physical miscue, especially if it's preventable.

As detailed in previous chapters, the number one way that you can keep yourself from getting hurt during your training is to keep track of any significant aches and pains that you may feel. Trust me, there will be quite a few of them, so make sure you make note of them in your training log. Describe the pain in detail, along with its severity and when it started. If necessary, you and your doctor will then have a reference to go back and determine when and how the injury began.

You should also review the use of proper, well-fitting running gear, especially when it comes to shoes and socks. Your body takes a tremendous amount of pounding when you run, beginning with the impact of your feet on the ground. Good shoes can make a huge difference on how sore you feel the next day and how fast you recuperate after long training runs. Also, don't forget to pick out a good pair of running socks in order to keep blisters away.

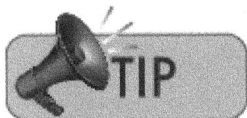

Here's a Tip! Don't underestimate the damage that blisters can cause. A severe blister, especially one that is infected, can keep you off your feet for weeks. Treat blisters immediately and do what you can to avoid getting them in the future.

There are a couple of other issues related to injuries that we have yet to discuss. The first is pain. Minor aches and pains are part of the process, but some pains are more serious, and you should know when it's time to worry or take additional measures, like seeing a doctor, getting treatment, or even suspending your training regimen. We'll discuss that next, along with how to prevent injury with proper stretching.

## Pain

Earlier in the book, I advised you (numerous times) to get a check-up with your healthcare provider before you start any physical training program. By now, you've done so and have started your training. However, now I must urge you to stay in contact with him or her, not only at the beginning of your training, but during the entire process. Remember, your body is a fine-tuned machine, but every machine needs a mechanic. That's where your physician comes in.

With the number of miles you'll be logging each week, minor aches and pains will be inevitable. However, it's important to keep minor pains from leading to major injuries. So, how can you tell when an ache or pain is something to worry about? I'm afraid that's up to you and your healthcare provider. It's impossible for me to tell you because I don't know your body like you do.

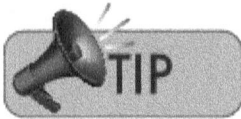

Here's a Tip! After you have your pre-training check up, make another "check in" appointment to talk about the aches and pains you know you will have. Schedule that appointment with your doctor, nurse practitioner, physician's assistant, or with a trainer. More and more clinics now have trainers on staff. They are a terrific resource you can use.

## Stretching

Stretching and warming up prior to running is extremely important, but not all stretching exercises are created equal. In fact, improper stretching can be just as dangerous, or more so, than not stretching at all. As my doctor has told me, poor stretching habits are the second leading cause of injury for runners, for both runners who do not stretch very much and for those who spend an inordinate amount of time stretching.

The key to stretching is to learn how to work every muscle group with long, slow stretches. I encourage you to do some additional research on proper stretching, as flexibility is a critical part of being a successful long-distance runner. You may be surprised to find just how more flexible you can become simply by incorporating a regular stretching routine into your daily life, on top of the stretching you do before heading out for a run. It is most effective when performed several times a week; however, a minimum of one good stretching session per week is sufficient to maintain flexibility for running. Many people stretch right away in the morning as part of their routine, which I think is a good idea in that you won't have to remember to stretch later on in the day.

Most experts and running coaches will tell you that proper stretching, both before and after your runs, will go a long way in reducing soreness. Gentle stretching after an intense workout also promotes faster healing and removes lactic acid from the muscles. After long runs and especially in the early stages of your training program, you'll likely feel a great amount of soreness the next day. Stretching before and after your runs will help reduce that soreness—and hopefully allow you to get out of bed in the morning without too many grunts and groans.

Make sure that your stretches are slow and gentle and that you hold the stretch. Bouncing into a stretch can cause more harm than good, and you'll be more likely to wind up with a torn muscle if you do so. If you've never experienced one of these, let's just say I wouldn't recommend it. A torn muscle will sideline you for weeks.

I often find that I am able to stretch better after I've had a short warm-up run. This is especially true if I had a long run the day before. In these situations, I'll stretch for a few minutes and run for a half mile or so. Then I'll stretch again. I find that my muscles respond better to stretching after they are warmed up.

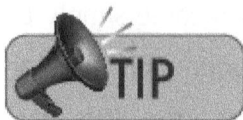

Here's a Tip! Do not stretch beyond the point where you begin to feel tightness in the muscle, do not push through muscle resistance, and never stretch to the point of discomfort or pain.

## Stretching Techniques

Always remember to stretch slowly and hold the stretch for 30 to 40 seconds. You should try to build stretching into your regular schedule both before and after your daily run. A good program should include stretches for the calves, shins, hips, buttocks, and thighs.

Here are some suggestions for stretches you can use:

### Wall Pushup #1

This exercise will stretch your calve muscles. With your feet flat on the ground and shoulder width apart, place your hands on a wall with your arms straight (you should be standing about three feet from the wall). Now, lean your hips toward the wall and bend your knees slightly. You should feel it in your calves.

### Wall Pushup #2

Keep your feet in the same place, and bend at the waist to a 90 degree position (hands on wall straight in front of you). Tuck your head down and look at your feet. Now, pull one foot forward with your knee slightly bent. Flex your toes up, and feel the stretch in the muscle below your calf. Repeat this exercise with your other leg.

## Wall Pushup #3

Stay bent at the waist with your head tucked between your arms; pull your feet together in the same spot (about three feet from the wall). Now, flex both feet up while rocking back on your heels. Can you feel the stretch in your shoulders, lower back, and hips? You should.

## Hamstring Stretch

Now lie down on your back (on a firm surface like the ground outside or the floor inside). Bend your knee and pull your foot toward your bottom until it is flat on the ground. Now raise your other leg straight up in the air. Loop a T-shirt or towel over your raised foot (in the arch). With equal pressure, gently pull down as you push away with your foot. Pull and push only until you feel your muscles contracting. Repeat with opposite leg.

## Heel to Buttock

Resume your position approximately three feet away from a wall. Place your left arm straight out with hand flat against the wall. Bend your right knee, and catch the bottom of your heel with your right hand behind your buttock. Pull your heel toward your buttock, get as close as you comfortably can. Repeat with opposite leg. This exercise stretches your quadriceps.

## Groin Stretch

Sit on the ground with the soles of your feet together and pulled as close to your body as is comfortable. Place your elbows inside the crease at your knees and hold your ankles. Slowly push your knees toward the ground; stop when this becomes uncomfortable.

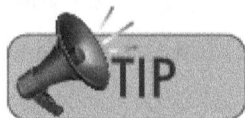

Here's a Tip! I learned this one the hard way: Don't trip. I'm serious about this. In researching long-distance running, I talked with three people who hurt themselves (one badly enough that she was not able to run her race) because they were in a runner's fog and fell. Pay attention out there.

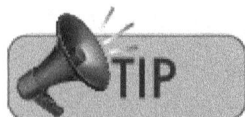

Here's another Tip! Your second long-distance event will be much easier and more pleasant than your first for one important reason: You'll know what to expect. This applies to your body, as well. When you're training for subsequent races, you will come to expect certain aches and pains at different stages of your training. Not only that, but you will get better at knowing what you can do to fix the problem.

Keep in mind that pain is an indicator that something is wrong with your body. Think of pain as a warning light on your car. If you have an unusual pain, think of it as a "check engine" light. Instead of ignoring it (like I often do with my car), go see your doctor.

# 10: THE NEXT TEN WEEKS

> *"Hard things take time to do. Impossible things take a little longer."*
>
> - Percy Cerutty

First, I want to give you kudos on making it to your first day of your training program. By now, you have completed your pre-training, considered a new way to approach your nutrition habits, have invested in some quality running gear and, let's not forget, you have had a check-up with your healthcare provider.

One of the things you may be expecting over the next twelve weeks is that in the process you'll have to log numerous 13-mile runs. Well, I've got some good news: the only 13-mile run you'll have to complete is on race day.

Now, you may be asking yourself how that's possible. After all, if you don't run 13 miles in training, how can you expect to run that far during the actual event? Let me explain. Although you won't be running that far in your training, you will know that you're able to do so.

Another thing I encourage you to do is to not think of the half-marathon as 13.1 miles at all. Rather, think of it as running a series of shorter races. By the end of the twelve weeks, you'll be able to run three miles, no problem. So, when you approach the half-marathon and your longer training runs, think of it as going on four easy three-mile runs. While you're running, only think of the three-mile portion that you're on, and you'll find the event to be much more manageable.

## Introduction to the Training Program

Just as you should break the race down into smaller segments, you should apply the same concept to your training.

Let's say, for example, that you can comfortably run a full mile. If that's the case, then you can run two miles. Then, after getting comfortable with three miles, you'll be able to run six. You see, throughout the training program, you'll be getting accustomed to running long distances, but distances shorter than 13 miles. If you're able to comfortably run eight miles in your training, you'll be able to run 13 come race day.

Before you begin this program, it is critical that you establish a running foundation. While you can get by with a little less, I think it is really important to be able to run, very comfortably, three miles at a time. You should also be running between three to five days per week, averaging between eight to 12 miles per week. Although you can run a half marathon with a less significant base, it's much less fun and a lot riskier than if you have a solid running foundation.

By far, the most important part of this training program—or any long-distance running training—are the weekly long runs, which take place on Sundays. Throughout the program, we add miles every week.

In order to be successful on your quest, you're going to have to conquer the "long run." These runs are hallowed weekend traditions that are despised and loved, feared and revered, bragged and complained about. For your first long-distance mission, the half-marathon, we're going to gradually work up to long distances, reaching a peak of a 12-mile run.

Just remember, DON'T CHEAT YOURSELF! The long runs are crucial to your half-marathon success, so don't skip any of them. Nothing will derail your plans faster than cheating yourself on your long Sunday runs.

On the weekdays, the distances will be much shorter, although they will increase over time, as well. Make sure you record all of your runs in your training log, along with how you feel, what you ate before and after you ran, how well you recuperated and (if you care) your time.

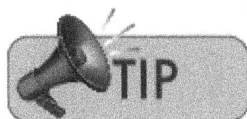

Here's a Tip! Take care in selecting your running routes. I like to find a route that is similar to the one I will run in the race, especially as it relates to hills. I also like a route that has drinking fountains or a place to stash water in bottles, and, ideally, at least one bathroom.

## Obey the Rules

Before your training begins, I want to discuss some ground rules that you should remember throughout the training process. The first has already been laid out, which is to get all of your runs in every week. The second, which is also very important, is that if something hurts, get it checked immediately by a professional. I know, you've read this countless times so far in this book, but I wouldn't include it so much if it didn't matter. I have a lot of experience with different types of injuries, and I'm hoping I can save you a lot of pain and suffering down the road.

Like I've said, some aches and pains cannot be avoided and you'll wake up many mornings feeling stiff. However, you know your own body and will be able to tell when something doesn't feel right. Get it checked out.

The third rule is that you should review the sections of this book on stretching and nutrition. Re-read those parts several times throughout your training and make sure that you're taking the proper safety precautions to prevent serious injury.

Finally, the fourth rule is just for you. Take a few minutes during each of your runs and be proud of yourself. Give yourself credit for what you've accomplished and look forward to the day when you finally run your half-marathon. You're on your way, and you're not going to give up!

## Cross-Training

If you look ahead to the grids I've provided for each of your training weeks, you'll be running Tuesdays, Wednesdays, Thursdays, and Sundays, with Mondays and Fridays off. You'll also notice that we'll be doing some cross-training on Saturdays. The type and intensity of your cross-training sessions will be largely up to you, but I'll provide you with some exercises that I've used in the past and have found to be effective.

For a variety of reasons, many accomplished runners incorporate a significant amount of cross-training into their conditioning routines. First of all, it's a great way to condition your body without constantly pounding the pavement. Alternative methods of aerobic exercise, like swimming or biking, will help prepare you for your half-marathon while taking less of a toll on your feet, knees, and lower back.

Secondly – and I'll be the first to admit this – running can become boring. Earlier, I gave you some "mind games" to help you out on your long runs, but even experienced runners sometimes find it hard to deal with the monotony. So, instead of making your Saturday just another running day, use it to condition yourself in a different way. Who knows, maybe you'll find another sport you'll enjoy just as much as running!

The point is that you should find some other type of athletic activity to do on Saturdays instead of running. Again, the suggestions I make below for cross-training are merely suggestions, and you should decide how intense your workout should be. However, don't be afraid to push yourself.

Now that you know how your training will work, you're ready to begin.

## Week One

The first week shouldn't be much of a shock to you, as we are just going to build a little bit on the foundation that you've already established. The weekday runs won't be much of a problem for you, and we're going to end the week with a healthy four-miler on Sunday.

For your first week of cross-training, try taking your bike for a spin. A six-to-10 mile ride should give you a solid workout for the day.

| Monday | Tuesday | Wednesday | Thursday | Friday | Saturday | Sunday |
|--------|---------|-----------|----------|--------|----------|--------|
| off | 2 | 3 | 3 | off | cross | 4 |

## Week Two

The second week of training is exactly the same as week one. Hopefully, by the end of this week, you'll be used to your four-mile run and will be ready to move on. Go for another bike ride on Saturday, covering the same distance (or maybe a little more) than last week.

| Monday | Tuesday | Wednesday | Thursday | Friday | Saturday | Sunday |
|--------|---------|-----------|----------|--------|----------|--------|
| off | 2 | 3 | 3 | off | cross | 4 |

## Week Three

This week we're really going to step it up and add a couple miles to your weekly total. You may have noticed that your second four-mile run, in week two, was easier than the first one. Now we're going to bump that run up to five miles.

During the week, all we're going to do is add a half mile to two of your mid-week runs. Also, you may want to try a change of pace for your cross-training. If you've been biking the past two weeks, do something different, like swimming. If you're in a standard size pool (about 25 yards in length), try doing thirty to forty laps.

| Monday | Tuesday | Wednesday | Thursday | Friday | Saturday | Sunday |
|--------|---------|-----------|----------|--------|----------|--------|
| off | 2 | 3.5 | 3.5 | off | cross | 5 |

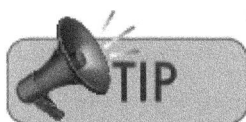

Here's a Tip! Use your days off (Monday and Friday) to relax and allow your body to recuperate. If possible, try to avoid strenuous activities on those days. It may also be a good idea to do some long, slow stretching on your days off to maintain flexibility.

## Week Four

Again, for week four, we're going to have a repeat of the previous week. This is so that you get nice and comfortable with your five-mile run.

| Monday | Tuesday | Wednesday | Thursday | Friday | Saturday | Sunday |
|--------|---------|-----------|----------|--------|----------|--------|
| off | 2 | 3.5 | 3.5 | off | cross | 5 |

## Week Five

It's time for another increase in mileage. Just as you got used to running five miles, it's time to conquer six on your Sunday run. Don't worry, you're doing great and that extra mile won't seem so bad.

I've also got another cross-training idea for you. Try doing some abdominal workouts on Saturday to strengthen your core. I recommend purchasing an inflatable workout ball. Not only can you do a variety of abdominal workouts with it, but it's also a useful tool if you have back problems, like me.

| Monday | Tuesday | Wednesday | Thursday | Friday | Saturday | Sunday |
|--------|---------|-----------|----------|--------|----------|--------|
| off | 3 | 4 | 4 | off | cross | 6 |

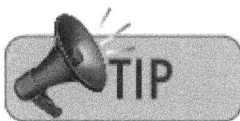

Here's a Tip! Start getting into a routine before your longer runs. I like to eat the same things before every long run, wear the same clothes for each long run, even say goodbye to my family in the same way before my long runs.

## Week Six

This week, we're going to increase your long run by two miles, bringing the total up to eight. Don't worry, you'll make it. Remember, you've already run six miles, which means you can run eight. Your weekday miles will remain the same.

How did the ab workouts go last week? Go ahead and do the same this week, or perhaps incorporate a little bit of weightlifting into your Saturday routine. However, if you're going to lift weights, make sure you check with your healthcare provider first. And take it easy.

| Monday | Tuesday | Wednesday | Thursday | Friday | Saturday | Sunday |
|--------|---------|-----------|----------|--------|----------|--------|
| off | 3 | 4 | 4 | off | cross | 8 |

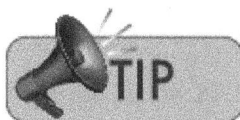

Here's a Tip! I tend to do my longer runs along the same route. That allows me to mentally prepare for longer runs, know where drinking fountains are located (or where I can stash water), and where I can get help or use a toilet, if needed. I know some fellow runners who like to run a different route each week, but not me. I like to know my course.

## Week Seven

Way to go! You've made it halfway through your training program. Didn't that go by fast?

We're really getting rolling now and are ready to bump up the mileage on both your weekday runs and your long run. Hopefully by now, the Tuesday through Thursday runs are not giving you too much trouble. On Sunday, you're going to go for your longest run yet at 10 miles.

Have you found a cross-training activity you enjoy yet? Don't rule out playing sports like tennis or basketball, both of which are great for conditioning. I've known a lot of runners who have been known to get together with friends and play racquetball once a week for a break in their running routines.

| Monday | Tuesday | Wednesday | Thursday | Friday | Saturday | Sunday |
|--------|---------|-----------|----------|--------|----------|--------|
| off | 3 | 5 | 5 | off | cross | 10 |

## Week Eight

After two consecutive weeks of raising your Sunday runs by two miles, this increase shouldn't seem so bad. We're going to add just one more mile to your long run and keep your weekday runs the same as last week.

Are you stretching properly? If not, refer to the chapter on warming up and stretching and you'll loosen up!

| Monday | Tuesday | Wednesday | Thursday | Friday | Saturday | Sunday |
|--------|---------|-----------|----------|--------|----------|--------|
| off | 3 | 5 | 5 | off | cross | 11 |

## Week Nine

You should feel pretty good about yourself, having completed two months of your training program with just one more to go. That being said, this will be your most intense week of running.

We're going to increase your total mileage by two miles for this week to 26, which just so happens to be about the distance of a full marathon. That's a pretty tremendous feat, if you think about it. You're a marathoner already!

| Monday | Tuesday | Wednesday | Thursday | Friday | Saturday | Sunday |
|--------|---------|-----------|----------|--------|----------|--------|
| off | 4 | 5 | 5 | off | cross | 12 |

## Week Ten

After last week, it's likely that you'll feel a lot of stiffness, so use Monday to recuperate. We're also going to back off a little this week with a shorter run on Tuesday and only a nine-miler on Sunday. This is still a fairly intense week of running, however, so be sure that you still take it seriously. After this week, we're going to start tapering.

| Monday | Tuesday | Wednesday | Thursday | Friday | Saturday | Sunday |
|--------|---------|-----------|----------|--------|----------|--------|
| off | 3 | 5 | 5 | off | cross | 9 |

When you're done with your nine-miler on Sunday, give yourself a well-deserved pat on the back. You have completed the hardest part of your training. It will only get easier from here.

# 11: TAPERING

> *"Human beings are made of flesh and blood, and a miracle fiber called courage."*
>
> - George S. Patton

It has been a rigorous ten weeks of training, but now you're ready to taper before the race. Congratulations. You've made it through the most difficult period of your training.

This chapter is all about those final two weeks. We will go over your program for those weeks and make sure that you're prepared both physically and mentally for race day. The most important words of wisdom I can give you at this time is to reassure you that you will make it. You've come this far, have completed the training and conditioning necessary, and are ready to take on the task at hand.

## Get Some Rest

For the next two weeks, it's extremely important that you get plenty of rest. This means allowing yourself to get a full night's sleep and not running more miles than what I've laid out for your training. Also, don't overdo it with your cross-training. Try to take part in activities with low intensity. Even a round of golf may give you enough exercise for the day!

Stay off your feet as much as you can, catch up on some reading or TV, and relax.

If you've missed a few runs over the last 10 weeks, want to lose a little more weight or want to work on a few more hills, now is not the time to make up ground. The best thing that you can do for yourself at this stage of the game is to rest.

## You Can Do It

Although the training program is going to be nowhere near as tough these last couple weeks as it has been, you may find things to be difficult for a different reason. You see, after more than two months of running, you've gotten used to your routine. While you rest, you might be longing to run and may even feel a little guilty about not running. It's also quite common in this stage of preparation for people to start to feel some self-doubt.

All you have to do is think back through the past 10 weeks. Think about how many miles you've logged and how hard you've worked. You are ready.

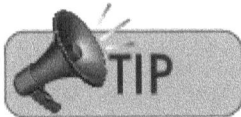

Here's a Tip! As you scale back on the distance and intensity of your workouts during the taper, you have to realize that you're not burning as many calories as you did during the more intense weeks of your training. Remember those pounds you shed in the last several weeks? Be careful in selecting foods to eat during this time period so you don't gain them back.

## Week Eleven

In training for a half-marathon, you have taken on an enormous challenge and are on your way to conquering it. Now, you might want to think about what's next. After all, if you've accomplished this much, imagine how much more you can do. Whether it's another long-distance race, such as a triathlon or full marathon, or something completely different, like going back to school or writing a book, think about it during your runs this week.

As I mentioned, this is where you start tapering before the race, so it will be a fairly easy week.

| Monday | Tuesday | Wednesday | Thursday | Friday | Saturday | Sunday |
|--------|---------|-----------|----------|--------|----------|--------|
| off | 4 | 3 | 3 | off | cross | 8 |

## Week Twelve

This is it, your final week of training. During your easy weekday runs, tell yourself that you're going to make it 13 miles. Take it easy during your cross-training exercises on Saturday, as you're going to need your energy for the next day's run.

| Monday | Tuesday | Wednesday | Thursday | Friday | Saturday | Sunday |
|--------|---------|-----------|----------|--------|----------|--------|
| off | 3 | 4 | 2 | off | cross | RACE |

After your run on Thursday, take a moment to reflect on your accomplishments. You have already conquered your goal of running a half-marathon. All you have left to do is to look forward to the race.

# 12: FINAL PRE-RACE PREPARATIONS

> *"Some succeed because they are destined to.*
> *Most succeed because they are determined to."*
>
> - Anonymous

As you approach the final two weeks of your training program, there are some additional preparations you're going to need to make to get ready for the big race. At this time, you may feel excited, tired or anxious, all of which are completely normal. After all, you have been working for months toward this goal and you are almost there.

This chapter will give you some advice on what you'll need to do in the final two weeks before the race to ensure that you're well prepared.

## Two Weeks Before:

Because you won't want to be worrying about details in the days or hours before the race, you're going to want to take care of logistics right now. This includes the following:

## Prepare Your Fans

Remember when I told you to talk about your half-marathon with your friends and loved ones as much as possible? Well, if you did a good job of it you're probably going to have some supporters who want to watch you run. This can be fun and motivating, but it can also cause a few headaches. You don't want your supporters distracting you from concentrating on your mission.

What I usually do is appoint my wife or a friend to manage my supporters. That is, instead of asking me details like where they should stand, they can go to my "manager," who will take care of the details for me. That way, I can give my full attention to the race ahead of me.

You'll also want your supporters to be scattered around the course. It will be nice to have people there for the final few miles, but it's also good to be able to see your friends and family throughout the race. Most half-marathons are run on a course that makes multiple laps, so your fans will be able to watch you run by multiple times.

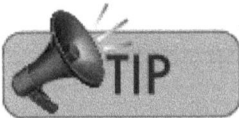

Here's a Tip! Know where to expect your supporters, but don't worry if you miss them. Also, don't slow down or stop and prepare to say a few words of thanks as you run by. Also, watch other people as their friends and family cheer for them as they pass by them.

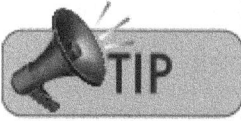

Here's another Tip! Your friends and family will think they are doing you a favor by offering you food and drink. Don't take it. If you have done a good job selecting your marathon, water and other fluids should not be a problem. Don't introduce new food at this late stage. You'd be asking for problems.

## Ready Your Gear

By now, you should have tested all of your running clothes in your long runs and have broken-in, race-ready gear. During your taper, wear that gear for every run.

Get your running fuel together and your sports drinks and gels. If you are going to carry gels while you run, buy several extra.

Many races will provide clear plastic bags with ties that you bring to the starting area. Before the race, you can put warm-ups, extra food and other items that you want at the start-line and will want again at the finish-line in the bag. These are things you don't want to wear or carry. Most of the time, the bag has a number on a sticker which corresponds with a truck or van number. Prior to the start of the race, check your bag and you can pick it up at the finish. I like to check my bag early. This gives me one less thing to worry about.

The worst thing you can do at the beginning of the race is to allow yourself to get cold. To avoid getting cold, I bring an old pair of sweats, two trash bags, an old hat and gloves to the start. I intend to throw all of it away at the beginning of the race, so I don't have to worry about checking it in.

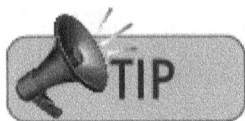

**TIP** Here's a Tip! Take off your sweat pants prior to lining up for the race. Especially in the larger races, the line of runners, even before the race begins, tends to move slowly toward the line. This means it's hard to remove a pair of pants after you've lined up. In most cases, your legs won't get as cold as your upper body, so ditch the pants and keep a loose-fitting sweatshirt that you can easily remove while you are running. I also like to wear a stocking hat for the first mile. I don't know if it really helps keep me warm or if it just makes me feel like Rocky. Either way, it works for me.

## Visualize Your Success

During your two weeks of tapering, you're going to feel like you have a lot of down time. Don't worry, the point of doing less running is to make sure that you're not worn out when you run your half-marathon.

Use this time to think about your success. Visualize yourself crossing the finish line. Think about the course you're about to run and what the scenario will be like when you finally complete your goal. Also, think about your friends and loved ones and how proud of you they'll be—or how proud they already are.

Make sure that you're eating well. Everything you put into your body will affect your performance on race day, so try to stay away from junk food as much as possible.

## One Week Before:

If you're like me, the week before the race you're going to be nervous. You may feel anxious and worried that you're not running enough. Just think of it this way—you've put in a lot of hard work and now is your time to relax and enjoy your time off. You <u>are</u> ready for your half marathon!

This week, try to stay off your feet as much as you can and don't go beyond the mileage we've set for your tapering. The few miles you will run are basically intended to keep you in the groove so you don't feel rusty on race day.

One of my favorite activities during the week before a big race is to catch up on movies I want to watch. I find this particularly enjoyable because it allows me to spend a lot of time with my family and keeps me relaxed. Whatever it is you like to do in your leisure time, I advise that you take full advantage of your off time.

### The Day Before the Race

Today is going to be filled with anticipation. You might be experiencing a little self-doubt, but don't worry. You're going to do something great tomorrow!

Do what you can to stay off your feet today. Don't run and try to walk as little as possible. Take a nap, watch TV, eat good carbohydrates, and drink lots of good fluids. Rest, relax, and enjoy life.

In terms of nutrition, be sure to eat carbohydrate products that have been "tried and proven" during your training period. Keep pasta sauces simple, avoiding varieties which are high in fat (e.g., alfredo, pesto, etc.).

Avoid eating a lot of salad items and vegetables (roughage), because these may prove to be troublesome on race day since they might tend to cause digestive problems. Stick to water during the evening meal. Because coffee and tea contain caffeine, these products may make it difficult for you to fall asleep easily. Caffeine (along with alcoholic beverages) is also a diuretic which can lead to dehydration.

I encourage you to pick up your number and other race material as soon as you can. Then, you can make sure everything is ready to go. Pin your number on your shirt and get all of your gear ready. If the marathon uses a "chip" to record times, lace it into your shoes according to the instructions you'll receive.

If possible, I strongly recommend that you visit the finish line today. More than likely, the organizers of the race are setting up the finish area. Go see it. If possible, spend some time looking at the finish line. Visualize yourself in the race running across the line.

Set your running clothes out, along with several layers that will keep you warm at the start line. I like to bring along a garbage bag that can be used as a raincoat if it's raining or in the event that I need a dry place to sit in the morning dew. Go to bed early and set two alarm clocks. Smile, you are almost there.

## The Morning of the Race

Treat this day like any other day. Go through your regular morning routine and make sure you eat the same breakfast you normally do before you run. Your spouse or family might want to make you a special breakfast for your big day, but try to avoid doing anything different. If you normally eat cereal in the morning, eat cereal today. The only thing you should add is an extra serving of carbohydrates.

Also take a few minutes to have some alone time with your spouse or significant other and talk about the race. This is a good opportunity to say a few words of thanks, and I find that my wife's encouraging words on the morning of race day gives me an extra burst of motivation. The feeling of someone believing in you can be a tremendous thing.

## Pre-Race

By now, it's completely normal to be nervous about the race. In fact, it would be strange not to have at least a small knot in your stomach. Have something to eat and drink some water between two hours and thirty minutes before the race. Stay off your feet, stay warm, and relax. You're almost there.

# 13: RUNNING YOUR RACE

*"There will come a point in the race when you alone will have to decide. You will need to make a choice. Do you really want it?*

- Rolf Arands

## The First Four Miles

You are now off and running. You're probably really excited and are feeling great. The number one thing to remember right now is to find your pace, just like in your long training runs. This run is no different from those you did in the past several weeks. Because you're so pumped up, you may have to tell yourself to settle down and find a rhythm with which you're comfortable.

If you're having trouble finding a good pace, try to find a pair of runners to run alongside or right behind. Two runners are more likely to keep a steady pace than a single person, so you might have better luck that way. If they are two slow or too fast, pick another pair.

Don't worry about your time—just enjoy the run. Stay loose when you run, keep yourself in control of your pace and remember to stretch your upper body every now and then and move your toes around. If necessary, talk to yourself to keep yourself calm. Remind yourself that you are making good on the promise you made and that, in no time, you'll be finished with your goal.

Above all, remember to get enough fluids while you run. Water is usually offered at the first tables at an aid station. When you drink, squeeze the top of the cup into a "v" shape to create a smooth delivery of fluid directly into your mouth if you choose to run and drink through the aid stations. If necessary, walk through the aid stations to be sure you are able to consume the entire contents of the cup. If you decide to stop and drink, make sure you're out of the way of the other runners.

Do not pass up any fluid stations along the way. For the first several miles, it's okay to drink only water, but runners must take in sports drinks before they hit 90 minutes of running. If you can, try to drink some sports drink well before this mark, however. Use your practice runs to find out what works best for you.

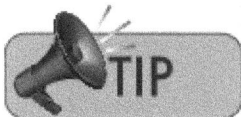 Here's a Tip! Remember to be careful of crushed drinking cups—they get slippery in the roadway—also watch out for discarded clothing.

## The Second Four Miles

You're well into the race and you're probably feeling pretty good. And you should be. You've run this far dozens of time in your training, so this should be no problem at all.

Staying hydrated should be your number one concern at this point. You also should have found a good, steady pace by now. If you keep a good rhythm, your second four miles will go just as smoothly as the first four.

Stay loose and stay focused. Things are going great!

## The Third Four Miles

Depending on how you feel, you may have to dig deep for this stage. Remember your long training runs and what worked and didn't work? Use that knowledge and keep your rhythm and pace. You should continue to stay focused (don't let your mind drift), and keep the fluids coming. You're more than halfway done. All you have to do is keep running!

Some people think this is the hardest part of the race, but not me — this is my favorite part of the race. During this part of the race, I like to look ahead at the people on the side of the course. I watch as my fellow runners spot their friends and family in the crowd and look for excitement on the faces of little kids. The atmosphere that surrounds these races is amazing, so soak it up and enjoy it.

## The Final Mile

This is the easy part. More importantly, this is the part of the race that you'll enjoy the most. Think of the last mile as your victory lap. Hear the sound of the people in the crowd cheering for you. You've almost made it.

I cherish the memories of the last two miles of my marathons. By this time, you know you are going to finish. Remind yourself how proud you are and how proud others are of you. Make sure you keep your fluids up and have a gel if you planned to have one.

# YOU DID IT!

Congratulations! You did it! You set a goal and ran your first half marathon!

After the race, you're going to want to sit down, but you need to keep walking. Even though your legs will be tired, it's important that you walk. When your friends and family come to congratulate you, take a short walk with them as a cool-down.

If your half-marathon provides foil blankets for runners after the race, take advantage. Otherwise, do what you can to stay warm. You're probably going to be really hot at first, but you'll cool down quickly, and you're going to want to keep your muscles from getting too cold too fast.

Don't wait too long before getting something to eat. Naturally, your body is going to be craving carbohydrates, but make sure that you get plenty of protein and electrolytes, as well. Sports drinks are good right now, even better than drinking just water. Grab some fruit and eat and drink slowly as you continue to walk around.

If you're dizzy, have severe blisters or another injury, or just don't feel right, get some help right away. Tell a volunteer that you need assistance and don't try to tough it out.

Keep walking and make sure that you're stretching frequently as you walk. Like I said, you're going to want to sit or lie down, but keep walking. After you shower, treat any blisters that you may have and make sure you keep them cleaned and bandaged. I use Band-Aid Advanced Healing bandages and New Skin Liquid Bandage. Also make sure that at this time, you stay off your feet for at least 45 minutes to an hour.

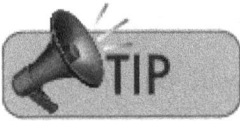

Here's a Tip! I'm not one to give parental advice, but I do want to encourage you to spend some alone time with your kids after the event. Again, you'll want to show them that you're fine after the race, but also thank them for their support and for cheering for you. Use your accomplishment as an opportunity to talk more about the importance of setting and reaching goals.

# 14: SO...NOW WHAT?

*"Well done is better than well said."*

- Gwen Haymore

As I've told you several times throughout this book, following through on a long-term and difficult goal, like running a half-marathon, will truly change your life. However, once you have finished the race, you may find yourself asking, "Now what?"

First of all, you should rest. The past twelve weeks, including the half-marathon itself, has probably worn you out. That's okay. Take a week or so, stay off your feet and relax. Also remember to continue to eat a healthy diet. Just because you've accomplished your goal doesn't mean that you should fall back into your old bad habits. Because you won't be doing any running this week, you won't be burning off any calories, so watch closely which foods you put into your body.

I recommend eating some solid servings of carbohydrates in the couple days following your race, along with soups, juices, and other healthy foods. Proteins are a good idea at this point, replenishing your damaged muscle tissue. If you're feeling restless, go for a walk and look forward to running again in the upcoming weeks.

After your week or so of rest, work your way back up to a solid running routine, with 20-to-30 minute runs the first couple weeks and gradually working your way up to distances with which you feel comfortable.

One of the things that you should be cautious of right now is avoiding injury. Your body is most vulnerable to injury after your half-marathon, so you should avoid running another long-distance event within a month of your half-marathon. If you are having serious pain that lingers for days or weeks after the race, don't hesitate to see a sports medicine specialist. Otherwise, take it easy and try to follow the advice given in this chapter to avoid injury and make a full recovery.

## Giving It Another Go?

After you run a half-marathon, you may feel pretty burnt-out. In fact, you may be downright sick of running. That's fairly normal. Take some time off from running if you'd like, perhaps turning to biking, swimming, or another sport for exercise.

However, many long-distance runners find that they can't stay away for long. This has happened to me virtually after every race I've ever run, where I go for periods with little or no running to months where I go out nearly every day. The choice is up to you. My advice is, if you don't feel like doing it, don't do it.

What's really important now is that you continue the good habits you've developed over the past several months. Eat healthy foods, get lots of exercise, and enjoy life to the fullest. Remember, you've done something that very few people have, or are able to do. Is there something else that you've always wanted to accomplish? Go for it!

## Final Thoughts

When it's all said and done, I want this book to be more than just a guide to running your first half-marathon.

In my first *Marathon Method* book, which outlined a training program for a full marathon, I said that running one is empowering. The same is true for a half-marathon. Hopefully, I have given you the motivation you need to take on the challenge.

Through the course of your training, you and I have been on what I hope has been a wonderful journey. If I've accomplished anything with this book, I hope you have been inspired to make your dreams a reality—whatever those dreams are. I hope you learned that if you set your mind to it, you can accomplish your mission. Most of all, I hope you are empowered and that you empower others around you to take chances, follow dreams, and take on their own missions—whatever those missions may be.

See you at the finish line.

Your friend,

Joe Donovan

# 15: ADDITIONAL RESOURCES

> *"Life is short...running makes it seem longer."*
>
> - Baron Hansen

**Running Clubs**: Some of the best resources available come from other runners. Talk to other runners and find a local running club. Weekly club runs often break up your training routine and can be a great way to meet new, like-minded people.

**MapMyRun.com**: This is a terrific website that allows you to plan your runs. Have lots of different running routes? You can store them in your account and use them again and again. This is a great resource.

**Runner's Word**: I find a lot of inspiration from Runner's World Magazine and a lot of useful information from the training sections. Definitely recommended.

Would you like to contribute other ideas for this section? E-mail us at:

ideas@marathonmethod.com.

# ACKNOWLEDGEMENTS

Writing this book gave me the opportunity to think about and thank all those who helped me run my first marathon, and whose constant support has allowed me to accomplish other goals, including writing this book.

**My parents, Joan and Jerry Donovan**, taught me the importance of competing, not to win, but in learning how to win and lose. These are lessons I am proud to pass along to my children.

**My older brothers, Steve and Dan**, have long been my idols, and I look up to them now as much as I ever have, if not more.

**My mother-in-law, Lonna Taylor**, has been to all of my marathons and is a constant source of support for me, Leah, and our children.

**My kids, Layne, Neave and Tighe**, are my cheering section. Their chants of "Go, Dad, Go!" help me put one foot in front of the other, mile after mile after mile.

**Finally, this book is dedicated to my wife, Leah**, whose calm reassurance and unwavering confidence in me and my abilities has kept me looking for challenges and following my dreams. I love you more than you can know.

# ABOUT THE AUTHOR

Joe Donovan is a business owner, father, husband, runner, and cyclist. Since running his first marathon in 1999, Joe has run three additional marathons and has completed a triathlon and several bicycle races. He is currently training for a long-distance mountain bike race and maintains the website, MarathonMethod.com.

Joe and his family live in Wisconsin.

Joe can be reached at joe@marathonmethod.com.

Published by Julian John Publishing,
a division of the Donovan Group Holdings LLC.

JULIANJOHN

www.ingramcontent.com/pod-product-compliance
Lightning Source LLC
Chambersburg PA
CBHW060552100426
42742CB00013B/2532